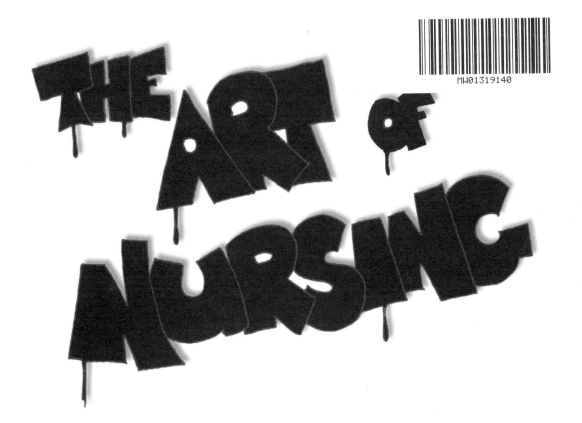

Nurstoons
THE ART OF NURSING

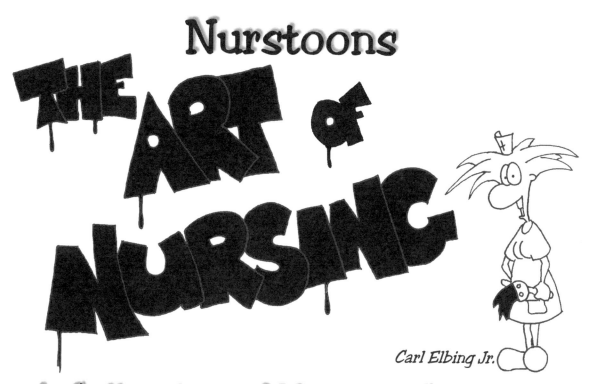

Carl Elbing Jr.

A Collection of Nursing Cartoons

Copyright © 2001 by Bandido Books

All rights reserved

No part of this book may be reproduced by electronic, digital or mechanical means without written permission from the publisher

ISBN 1-929693-13-3

For copyright clearance and to purchase Nurstoon products, please visit us at www.bandidobooks.com or contact us by email at publish@bandidobooks.com

Bandido Books 9806 Heaton Court, Orlando, FL 32817

Happy Nursing!

Printed in Canada

Foreword

Learned theorists say that Nursing is both a science and an art. It is a science because of words like microgram and oophorectomy (trust me, that's how you spell it). It is an art because, well, it takes a lot of creativity to pass out all 0900 meds at 0900 (and a bit of time traveling too). Only a Nurse is professionally prepared to wipe bottoms and differentiate v-tach from supraventricular tachycardia. Only a Nurse performs services, many of them lifesaving, which get billed as a room charge. Only a Nurse.

This book celebrates our profession in all of its irony, and it illustrates that *satire can be a from of care*. Enjoy this humorous look at the *The Art of Nursing*.

Martin Schiavenato RN
Editor
Bandido Books

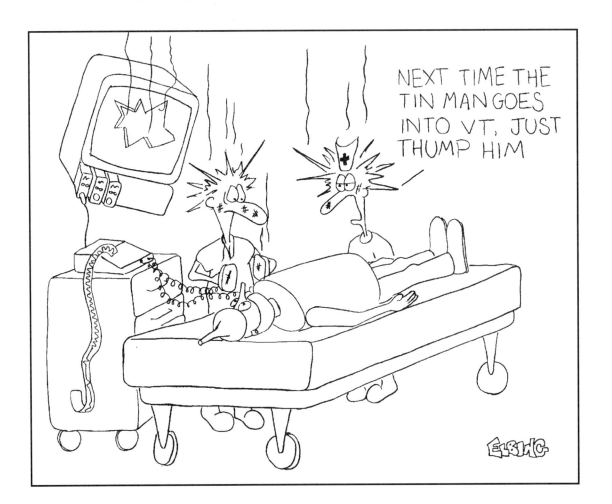

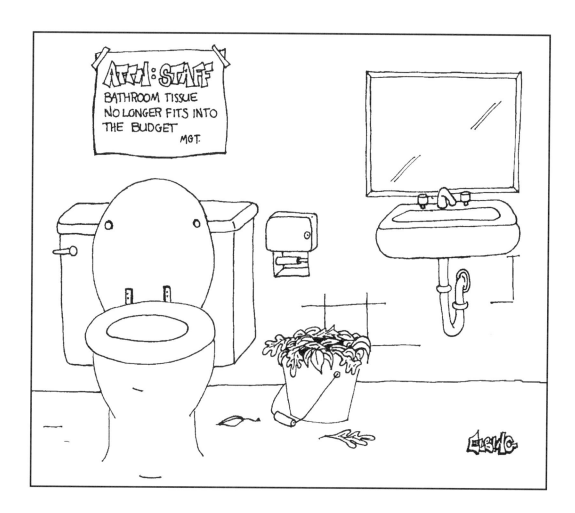

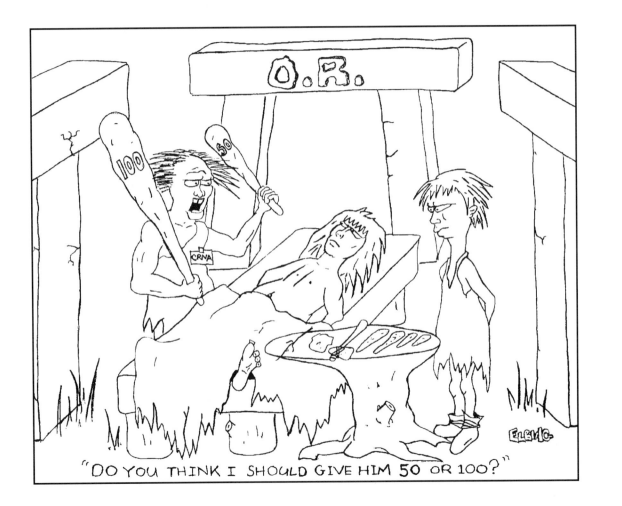

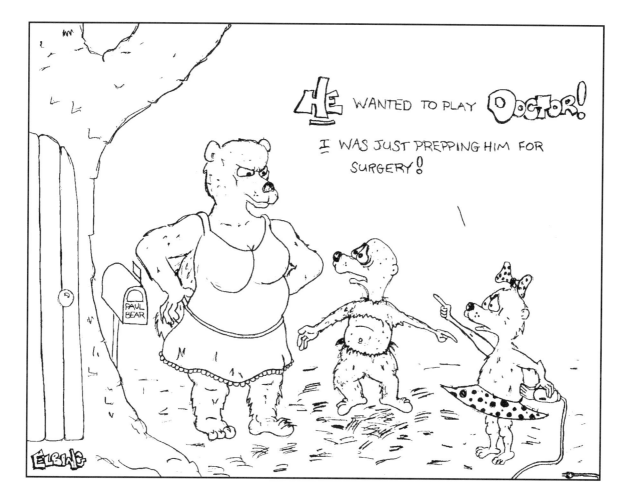

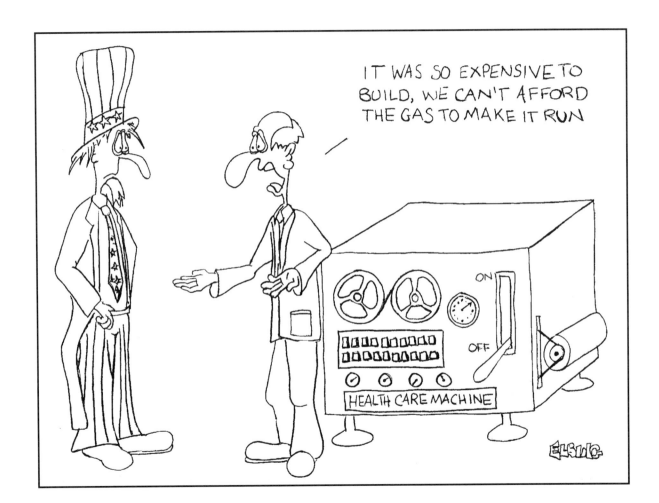

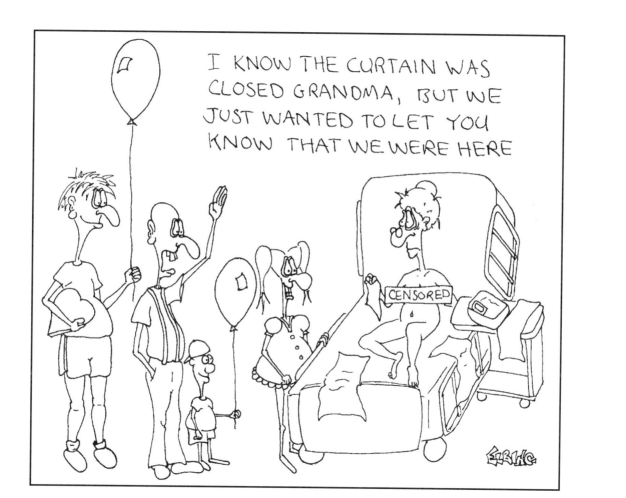

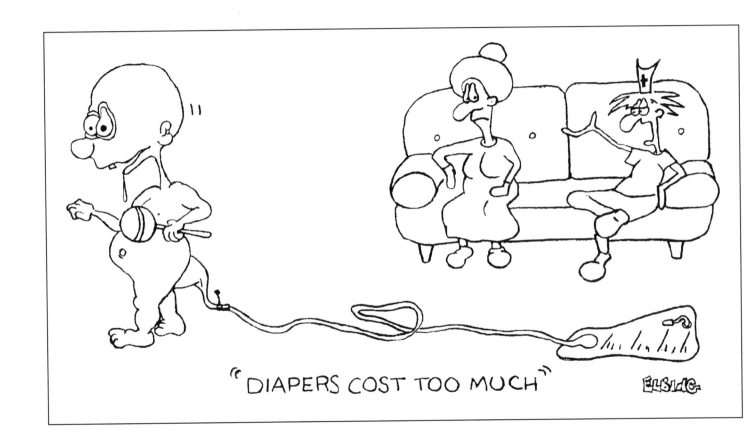

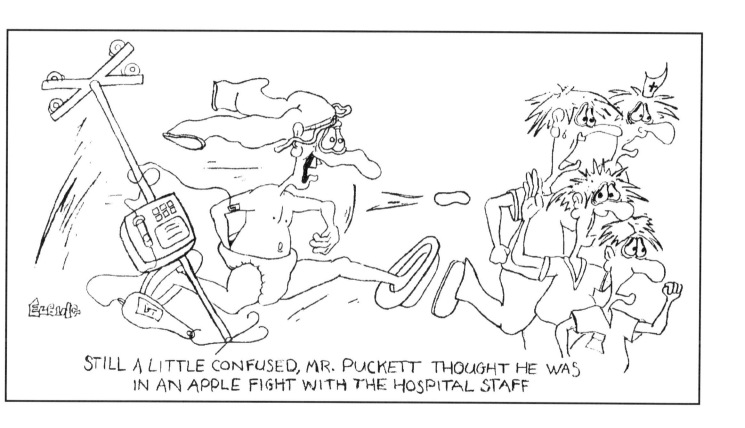

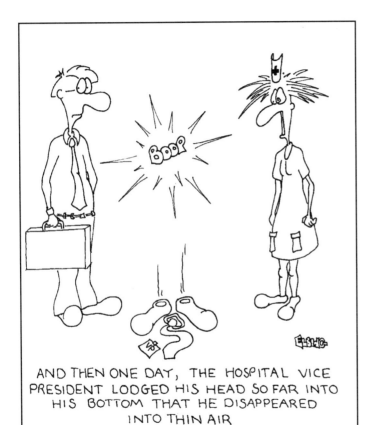
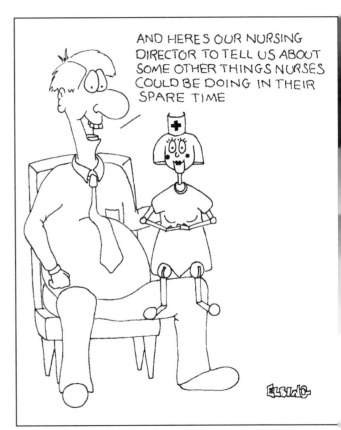

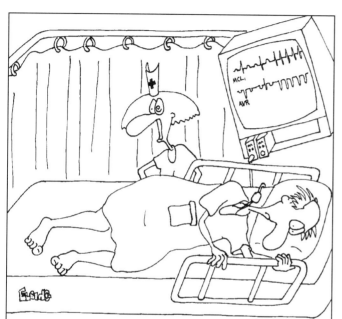
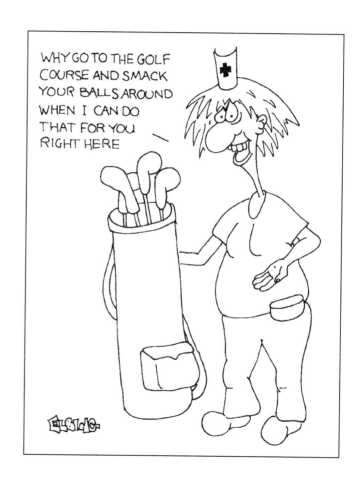

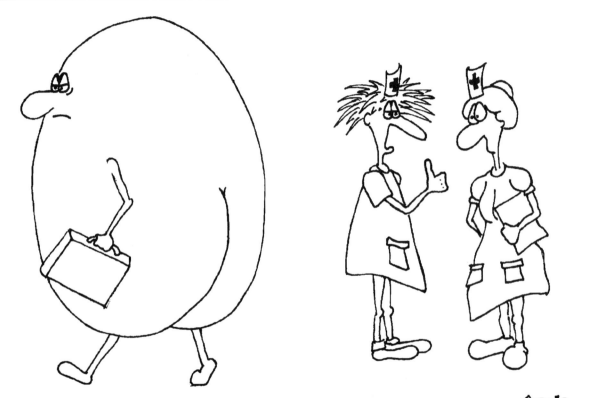

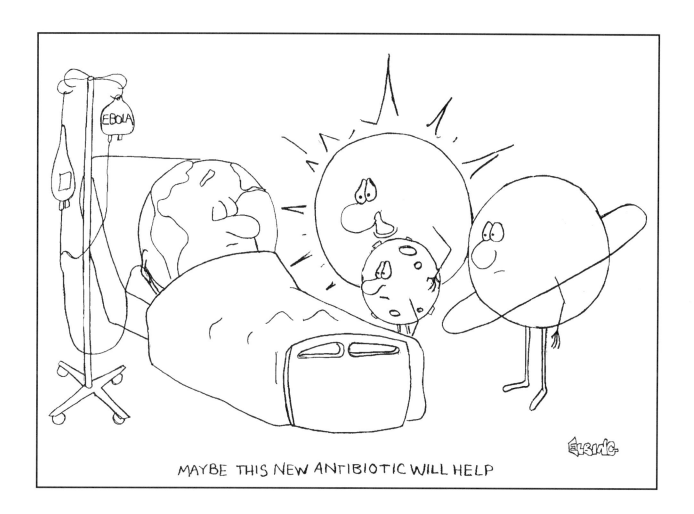

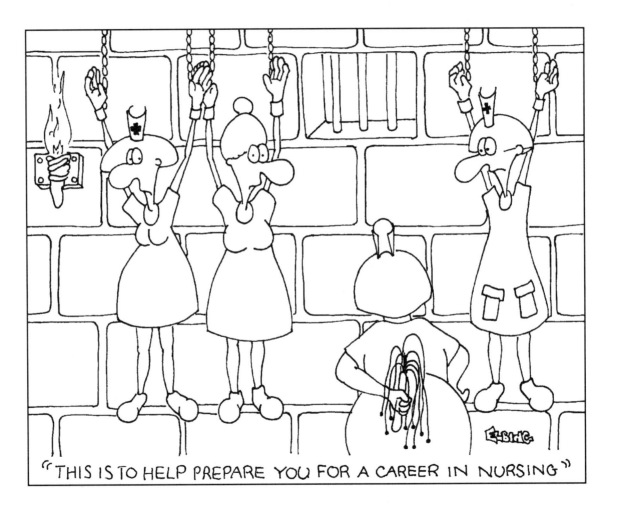

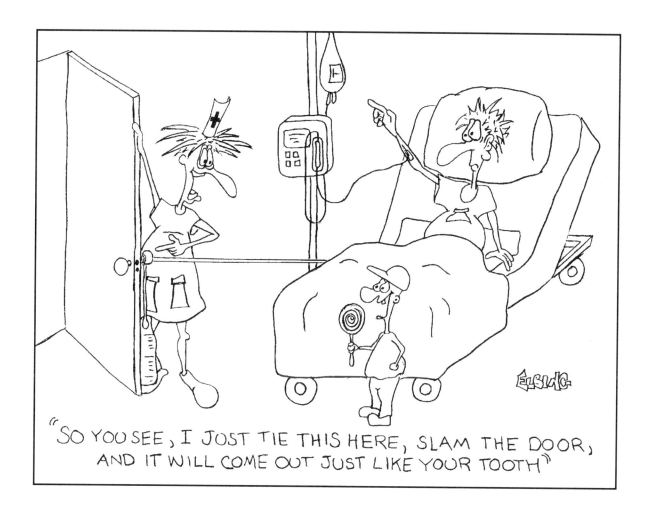

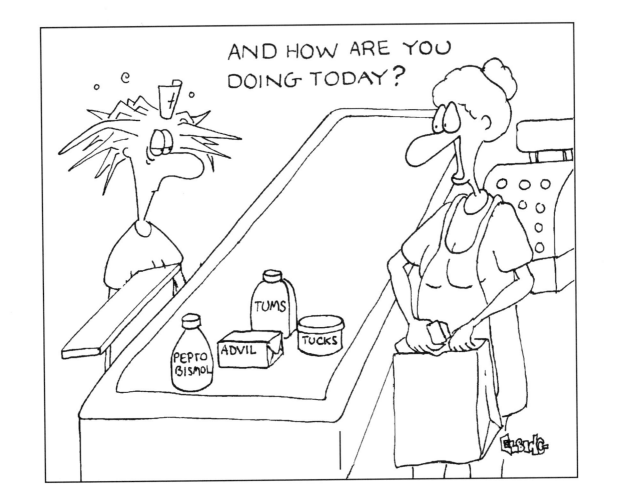

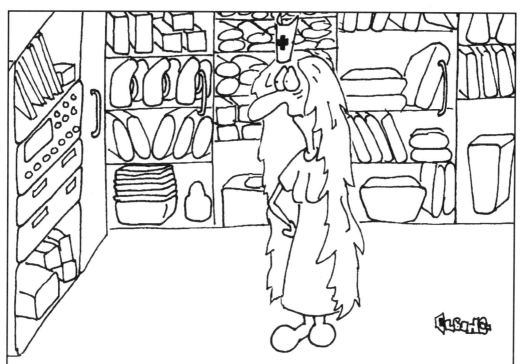

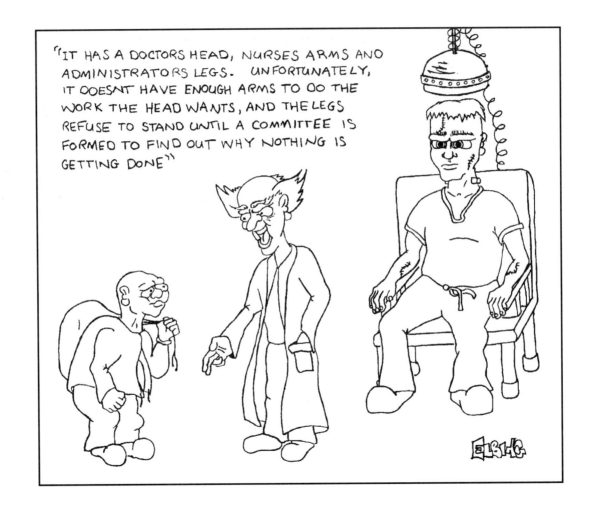

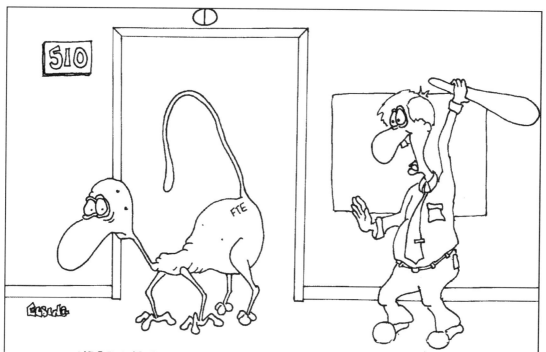

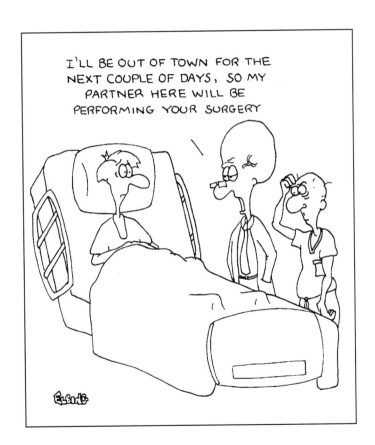 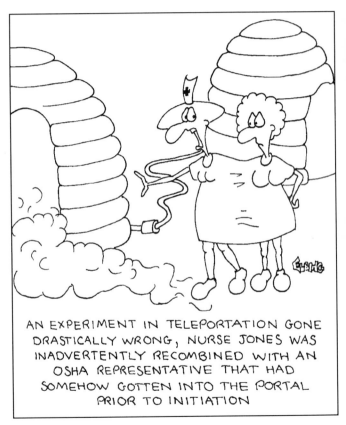

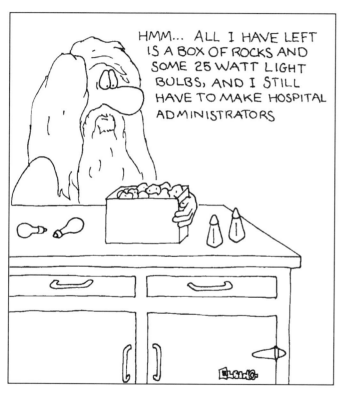

GODS KITCHEN

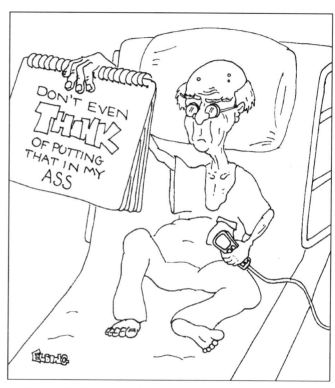

PATIENT DESIGNED COMMUNICATION BOARDS

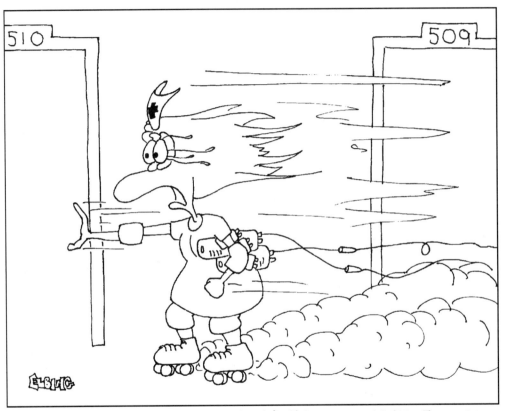

AFTER BEING SHOT FROM A CANNON, NURSE JONES WAS FINALLY ABLE TO DELIVER ALL OF HER 0900 MEDS ON TIME.

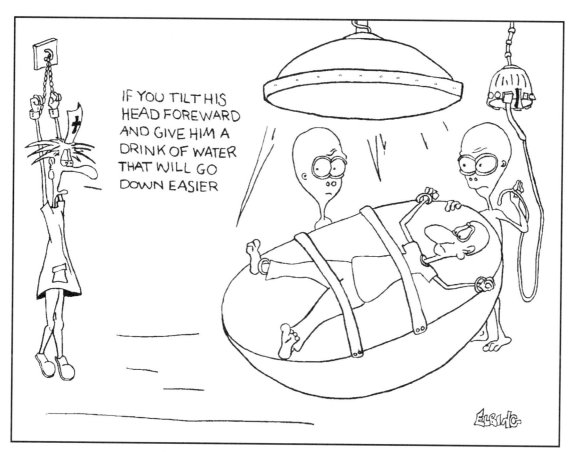

ONCE UPON AN ABDUCTION

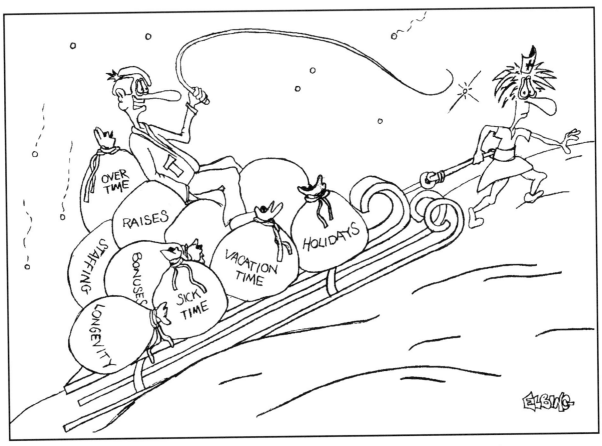

THE HOSPITAL VICE PRESIDENT WHO STOLE CHRISTMAS

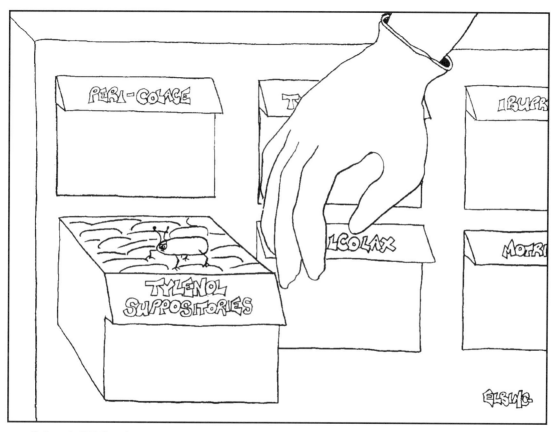

JUST HAPPENING TO BE IN THE WRONG PLACE AT THE WRONG TIME THE SILVER BULLET BUG INADVERTENTLY SEALED ITS OWN DOOM

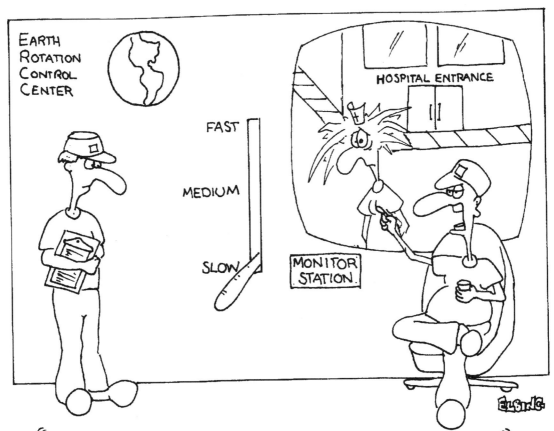

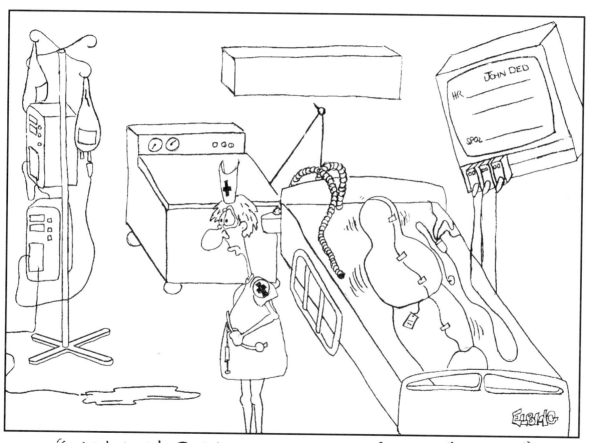

"NO! NO! I SAID WRAP THE "DEAD" GUY!"

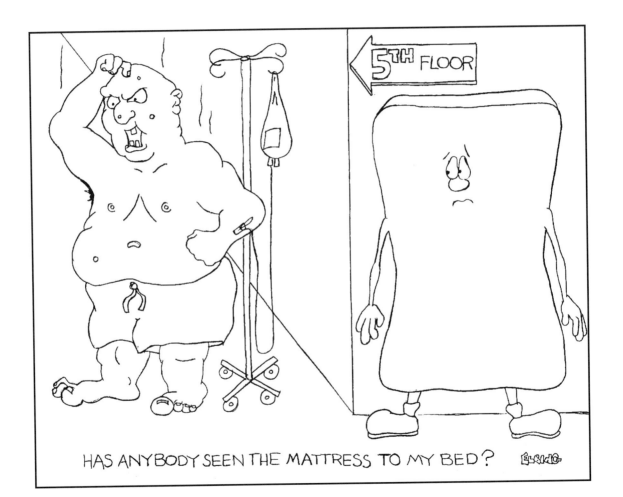

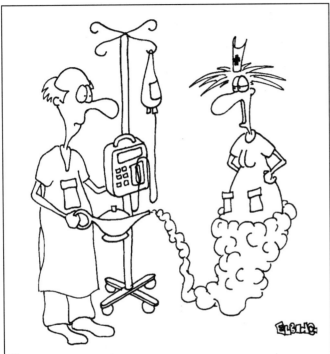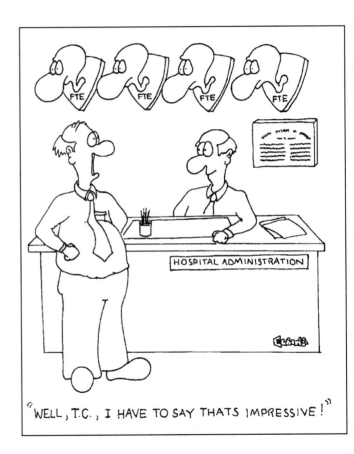

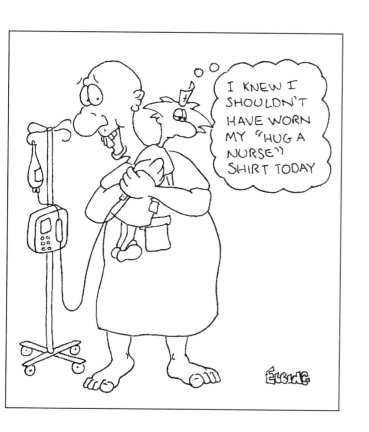

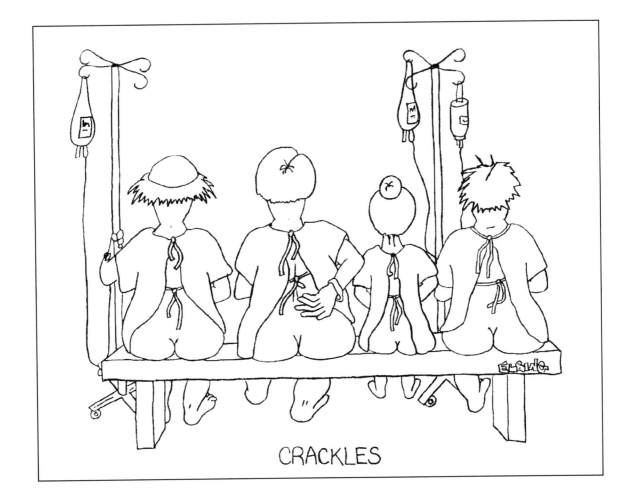

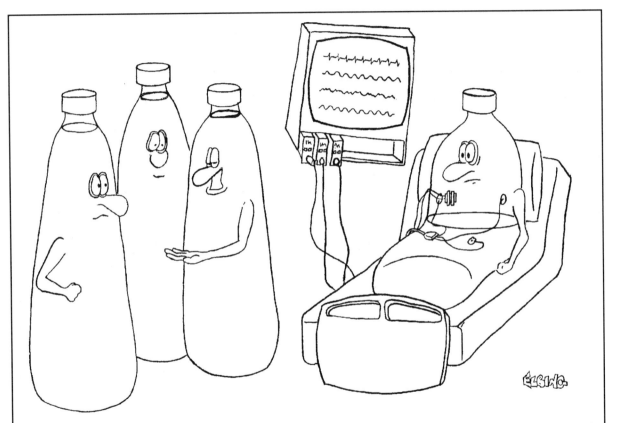

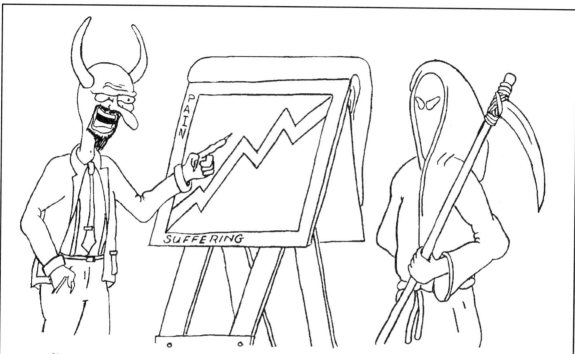

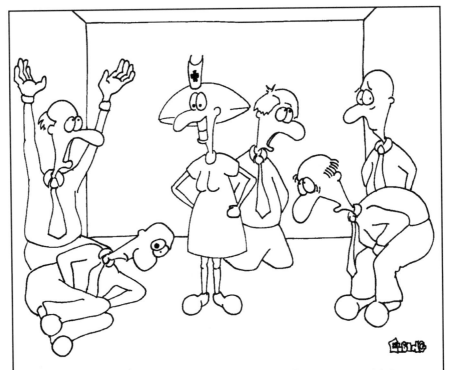

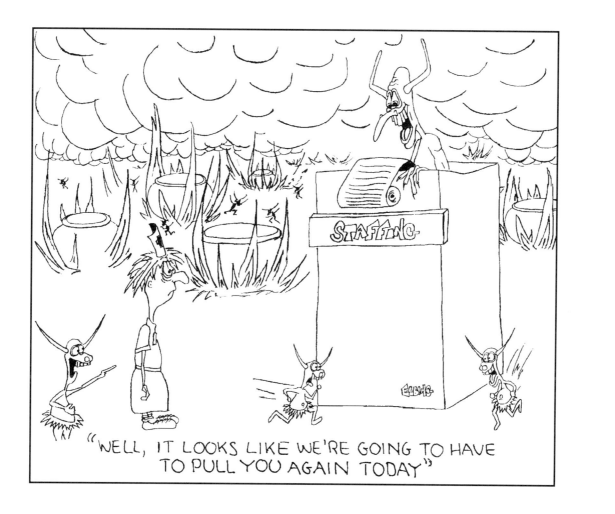

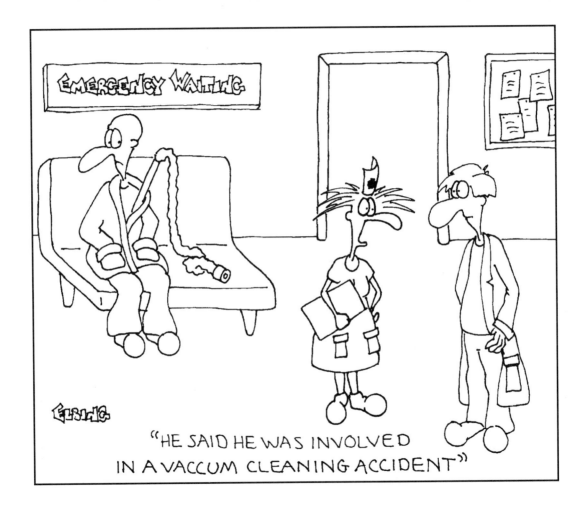

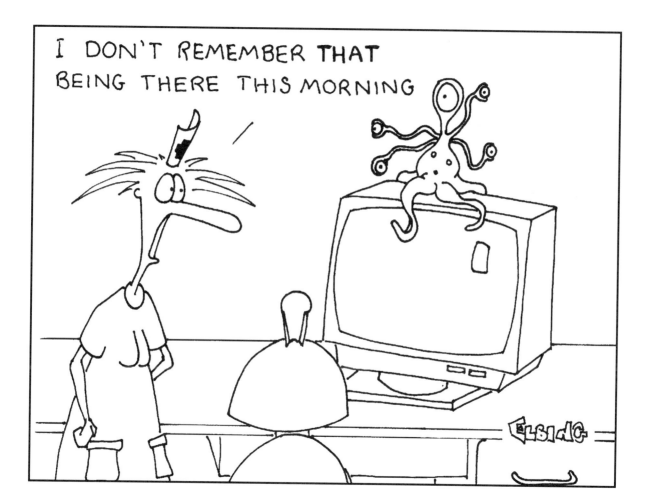

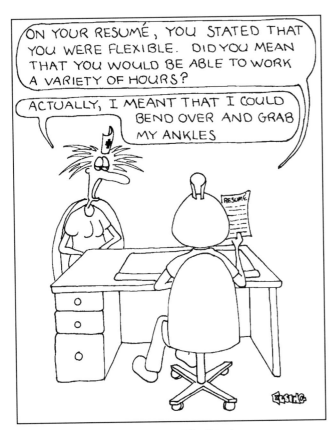

THE INTERVIEW

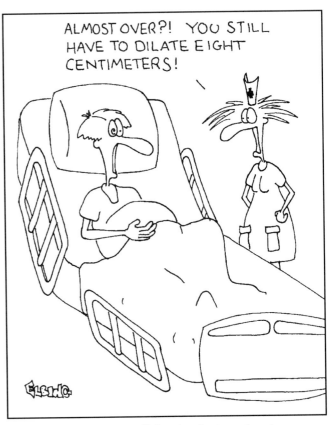

THE FIRST PREGNANT MAN

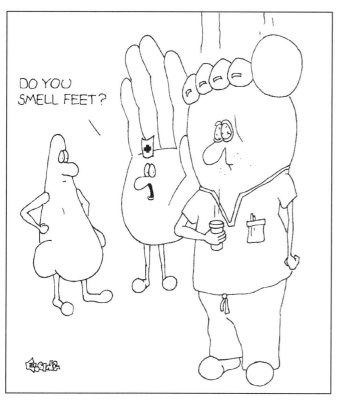

AFTER 36 HOURS OF BEING ON CALL...

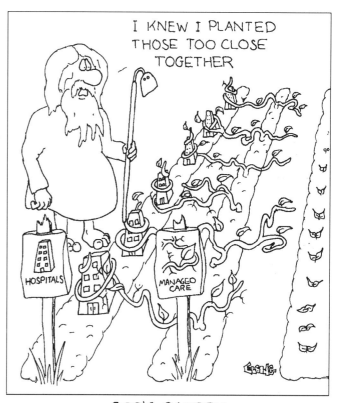

GOD'S GARDEN

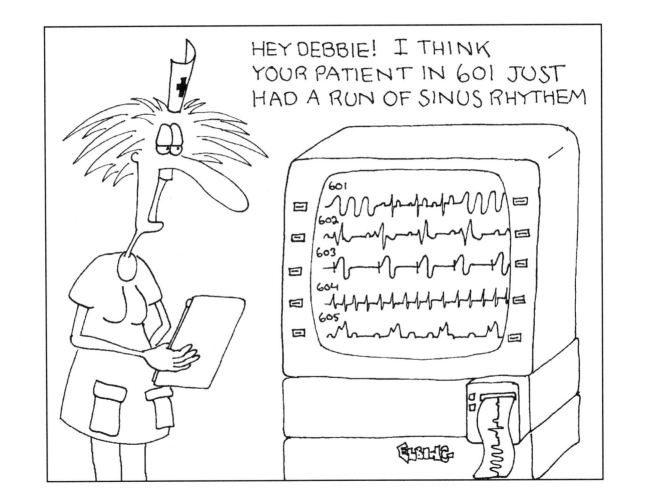

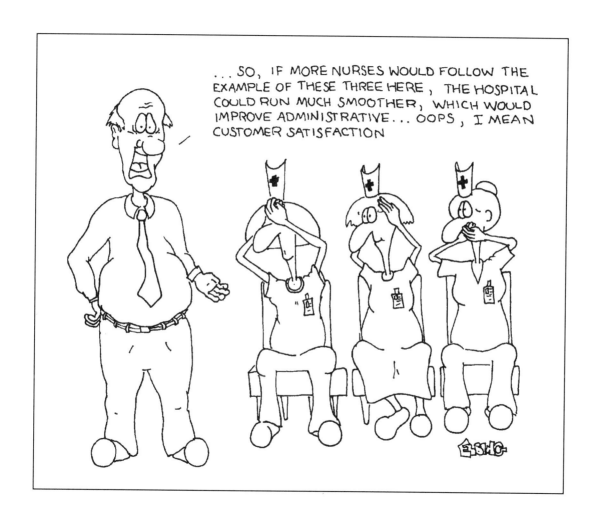

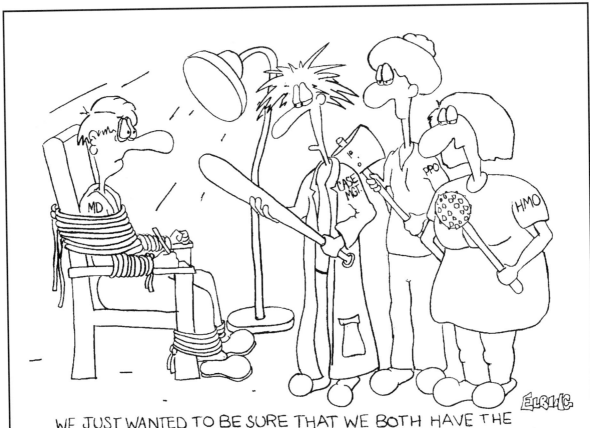

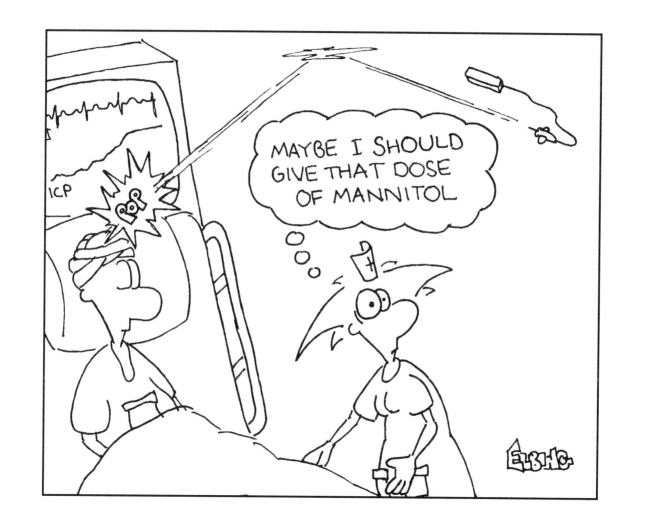

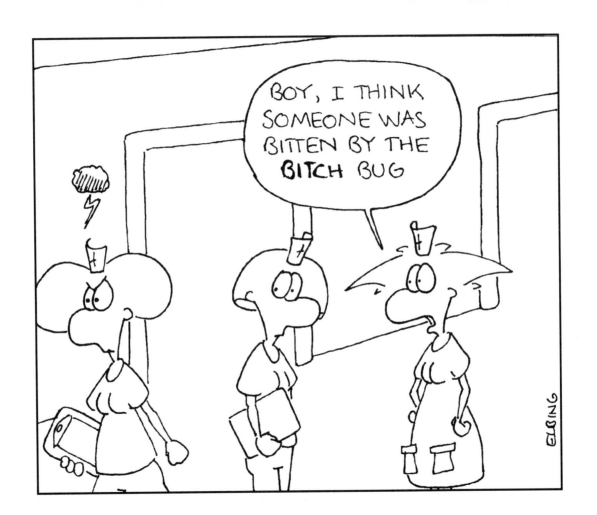

"AND BEHIND DOOR NUMBER ONE YOU GET A G.I. BLEEDER! BUT THAT'S NOT ALL! HE HAS COPD, CHF, RENAL INSUFFICIENCY AND HAS AN ENDOSCOPY AT 10:00! AND IF THAT ISN'T ENOUGH TO EXCITE YOU, YOU ALSO GET..."

REPORT GETS OUT OF HAND

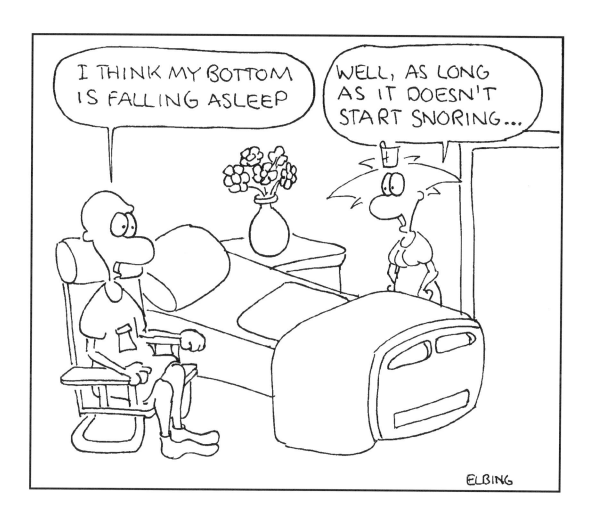

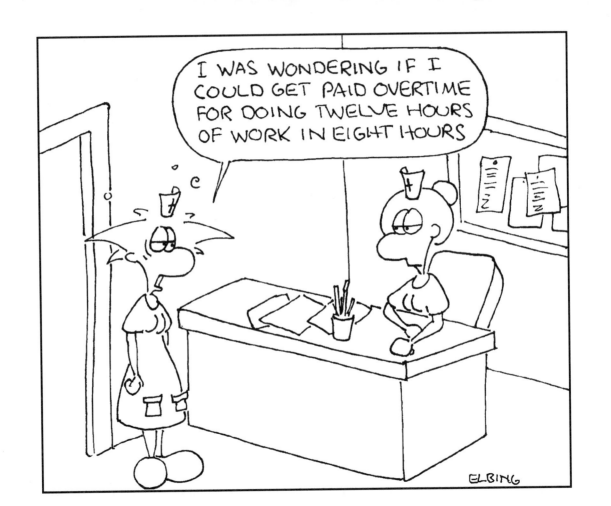

> I THINK THAT IF WE LOOSEN A FEW SCREWS, WE COULD CONVINCE IT TO WORK AS A STAFF NURSE

THE FIRST NURSE CYBORG

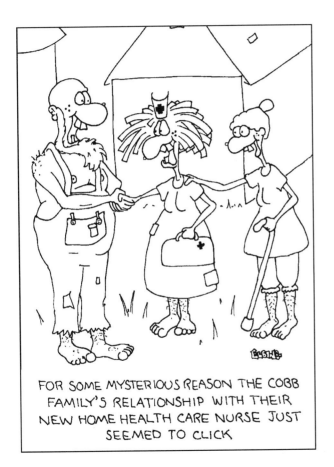
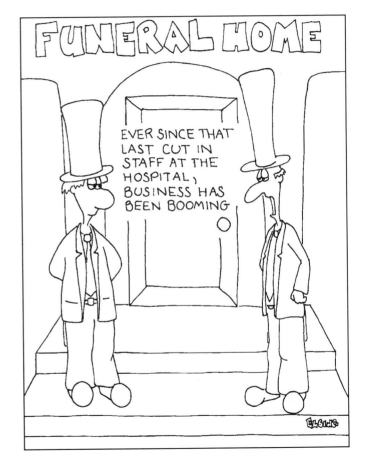

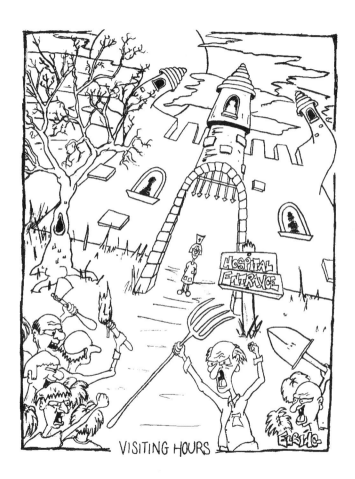

VISITING HOURS

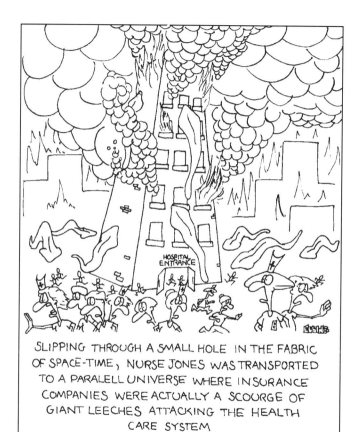

SLIPPING THROUGH A SMALL HOLE IN THE FABRIC OF SPACE-TIME, NURSE JONES WAS TRANSPORTED TO A PARALELL UNIVERSE WHERE INSURANCE COMPANIES WERE ACTUALLY A SCOURGE OF GIANT LEECHES ATTACKING THE HEALTH CARE SYSTEM

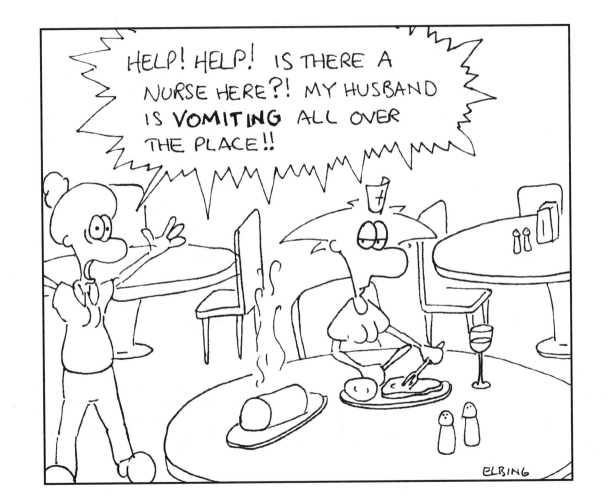

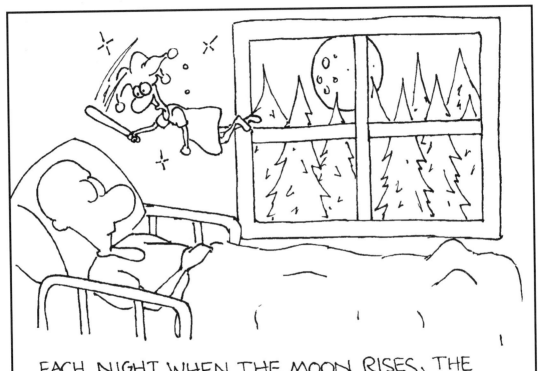

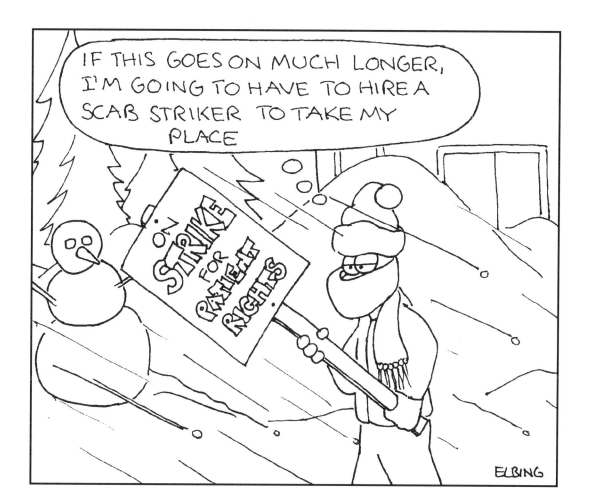

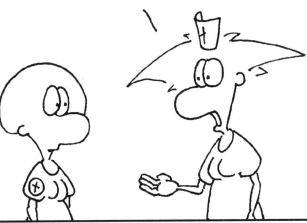

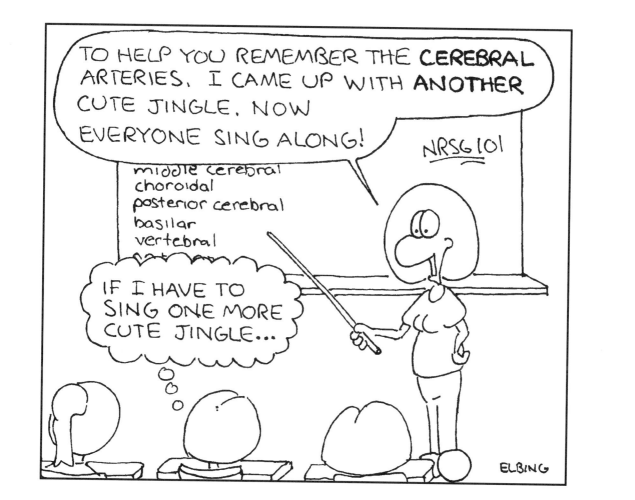

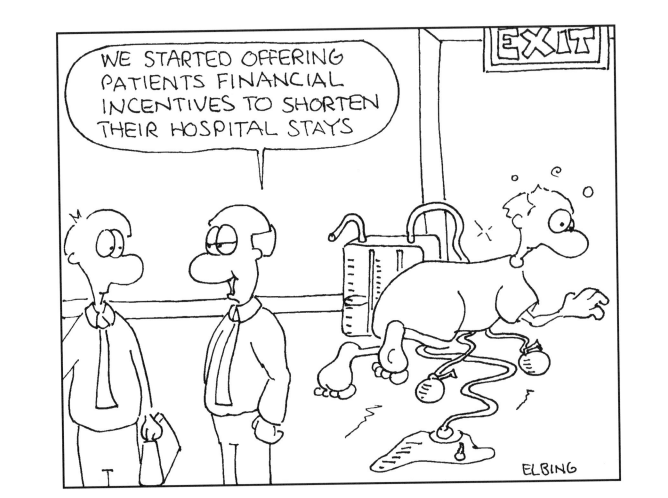

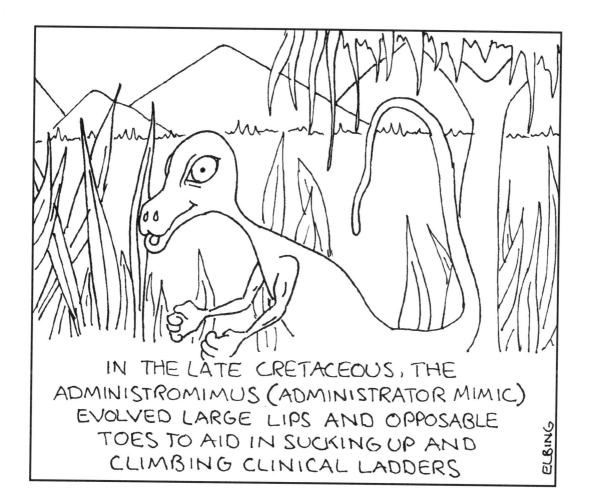

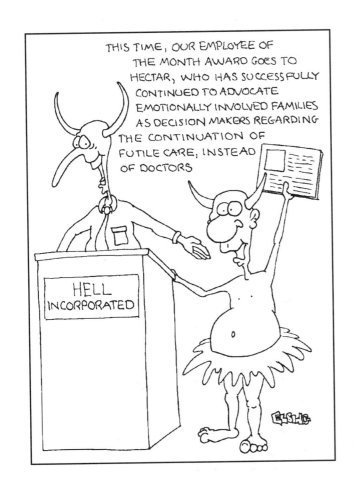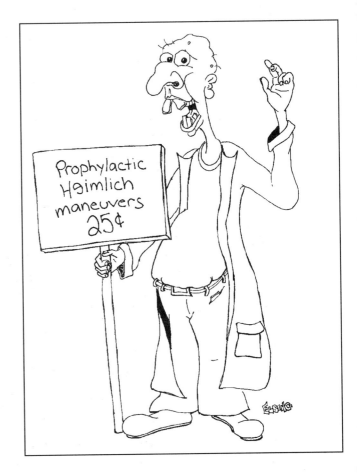

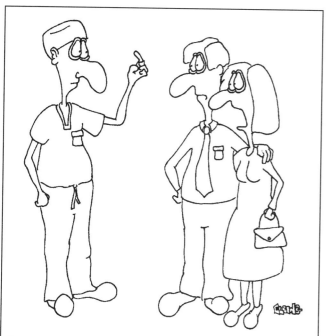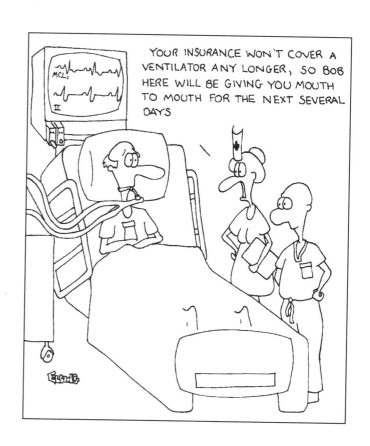

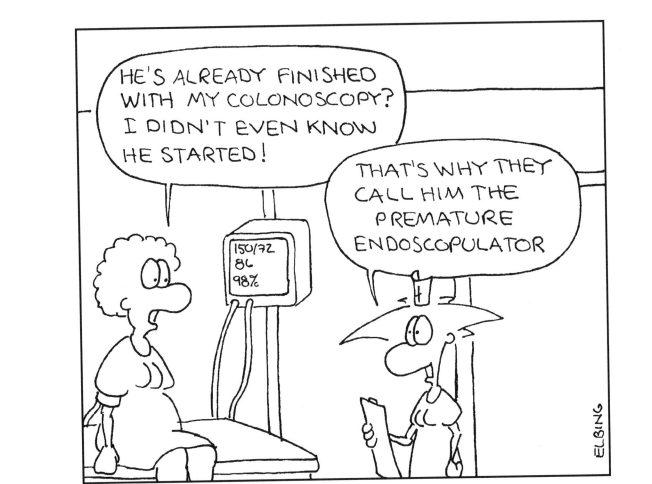

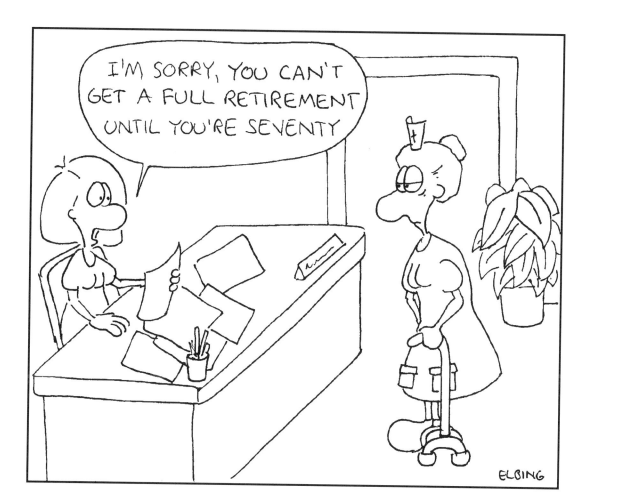

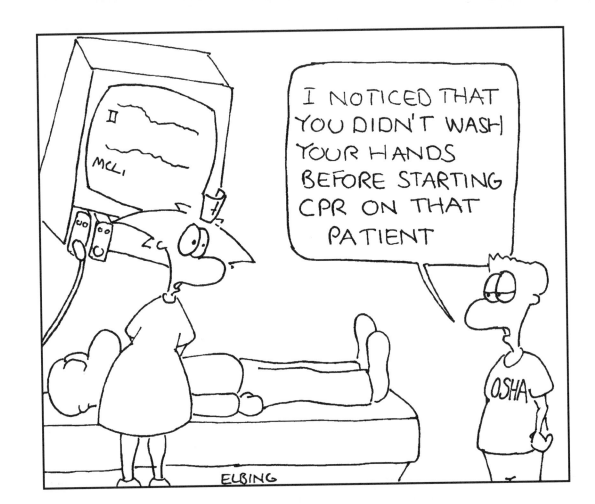

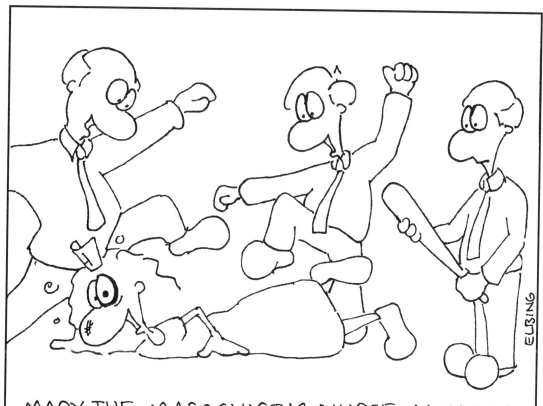

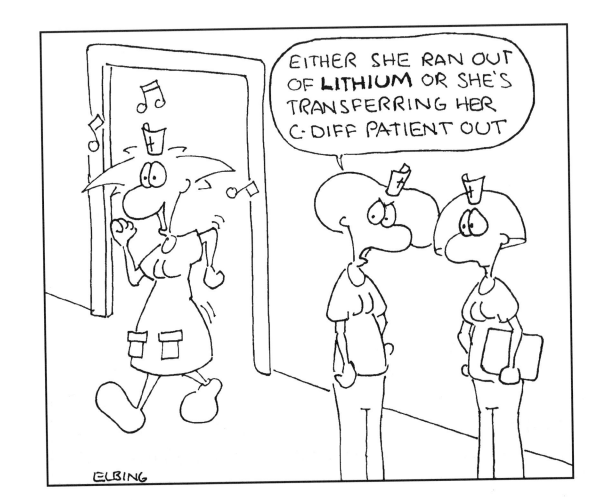

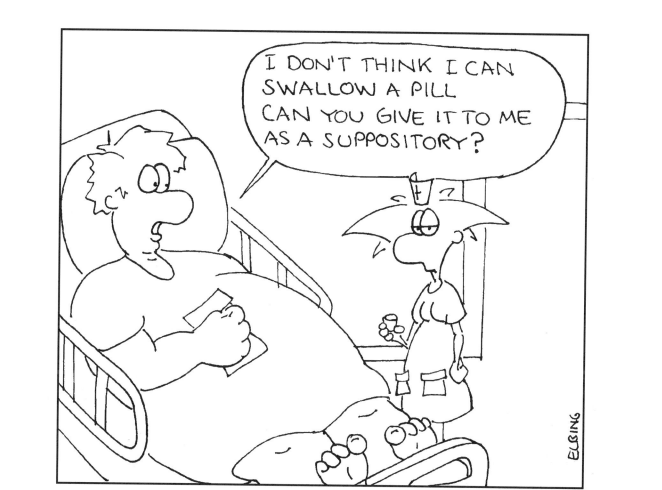

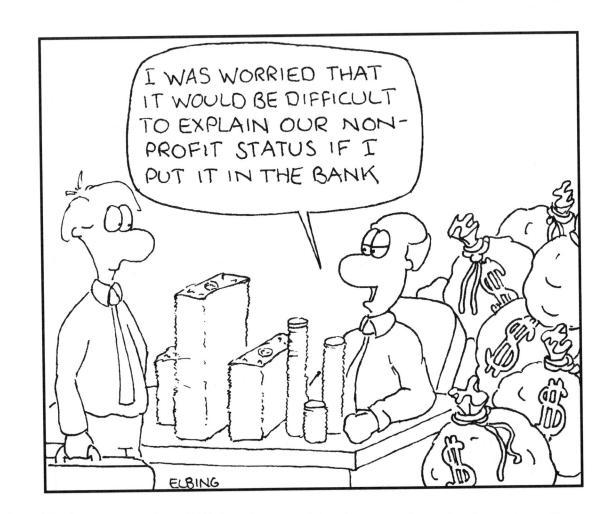

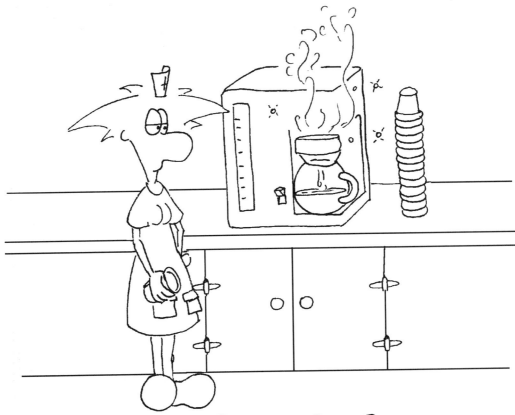

The End

About the Author

Carl Elbing is a working, time-card punching ICU RN who started publishing cartoons back in 1994. This is both an expression of his professional experience, and a required part of his supervised therapy. His sincerest hope is that his satire and lightheartedness help to shed a light at the pressing issues in health care today. He also would like to be allowed to hold the narcotic keys again.